Title: Baking Bread 101: Easy Instructions To Bake Bread From Scratch...

Table of Contents...

Welcome to "Baking Bread 101: Easy Instructions To Bake Bread From Scratch." This comprehensive guide is designed to take you on a journey through the art and science of bread making. Whether you're a novice or an experienced baker, this book will equip you with the knowledge and skills needed to produce a wide array of delicious, freshly baked breads right in your own kitchen....

In the following chapters, we will delve into the intricacies of bread making, covering everything from selecting the finest ingredients to mastering advanced techniques. Each chapter is meticulously crafted to provide you with in-depth educational content, ensuring that you not only learn how to bake bread but also understand the underlying principles that govern the process....

Chapter 1: The Basics of Bread Making...

Bread making is a centuries-old tradition that combines simple ingredients to create a staple food enjoyed by people worldwide. Understanding the fundamentals is crucial for achieving consistent and exceptional results in your baking endeavors....

Ingredients...

The primary ingredients in bread making are flour, water, yeast, and salt. Each plays a vital role in the final product, contributing to flavor, texture, and structure....

Flour...

The choice of flour is a critical factor in bread making. Different types of flour, such as all-purpose, bread, whole wheat, and specialty flours, yield distinct characteristics in the finished loaf. Understanding their properties empowers you to select the right flour for your desired outcome....

Water...

Water activates the yeast and forms the dough's structure. The temperature of the water influences the fermentation process and the final texture of the bread....

Yeast...

Yeast is a microorganism that ferments the dough, producing

carbon dioxide gas and alcohol.
This process leavens the bread,
creating a light and airy texture....

Salt...

Salt enhances flavor and regulates
yeast activity. It also strengthens
the dough's structure, resulting in
a well-textured loaf....

Mixing and Kneading...

The process of mixing and
kneading develops the dough's
gluten structure, which gives the
bread its characteristic chewiness
and structure. Proper technique
and timing are crucial at this
stage....

Mixing...

During mixing, the flour, water, yeast, and salt are combined to form a cohesive dough. This initial integration sets the foundation for further development....

Kneading...

Kneading involves a rhythmic motion of folding, pressing, and turning the dough. This action aligns the gluten strands, allowing the dough to rise properly....

Fermentation...

Fermentation is the magical transformation of the dough, where yeast consumes sugars and produces carbon dioxide. This process imparts flavor and texture to the bread....

Bulk Fermentation...

The first rise, known as bulk fermentation, allows the dough to develop flavor and structure. Patience during this stage is rewarded with a more flavorful loaf....

Final Proofing...

After shaping, the dough undergoes final proofing, where it gains its final volume and texture. This step ensures a light and airy crumb....

By mastering the basics of bread making, you are setting the stage for a rewarding and delicious baking experience. In the following chapters, we will explore each element in greater detail, equipping you with the knowledge and skills to create a wide range of bread varieties....

Chapter 2: Types of Flour and Their Effects...

Selecting the right type of flour is a crucial step in achieving the desired texture and flavor in your bread. Each variety brings its own unique characteristics to the table....

All-Purpose Flour...

This versatile flour is a staple in many kitchens. It strikes a balance between protein content and starch, making it suitable for a wide range of baked goods, including bread, cakes, and pastries. All-purpose flour produces a tender crumb and a mild, well-rounded flavor....

Bread Flour...

Specifically formulated for bread making, this flour has a higher protein content than all-purpose flour. The additional protein provides structure and elasticity to the dough, resulting in a chewier and more substantial loaf. It is ideal for hearty bread varieties and artisanal loaves....

Whole Wheat Flour...

Made from the entire wheat kernel, whole wheat flour is rich in fiber and nutrients. It imparts a nutty flavor and a denser texture to bread. Due to its higher fiber content, dough made with whole wheat flour may require additional hydration and longer fermentation times....

Specialty Flours...

Specialty flours, such as rye, spelt, and barley, offer unique flavors and textures to your bread. Experimenting with these alternative grains can lead to distinctive and flavorful creations. Keep in mind that these flours may require adjustments in hydration and mixing techniques....

Gluten-Free Alternatives...

For those with gluten sensitivities or allergies, a variety of gluten-free flours, including rice flour, almond flour, and coconut flour, can be used to create bread-like textures. These alternative flours may require the addition of binding agents and extra attention to hydration levels....

Understanding the characteristics of different flours empowers you to make informed choices when crafting your bread recipes. Experimenting with various flour combinations can lead to personalized and uniquely flavorful loaves....

Chapter 3: Yeast: The Heart of Bread...

Yeast is the unsung hero of bread making, responsible for the rise and flavor of your loaves. Understanding its role and how to work with it is key to successful bread baking....

Types of Yeast...

There are three main types of yeast used in bread making:...

Active Dry Yeast...

This granulated form of yeast requires activation in warm water before use. It provides a steady and reliable rise, making it a popular choice for many bread recipes....

Instant Yeast...

Also known as rapid-rise or quick-rise yeast, this type does not require activation and can be mixed directly with dry ingredients. It provides a faster rise and is well-suited for busy bakers....

Fresh Yeast...

Compressed into cakes, fresh yeast offers a rapid rise and imparts a distinct flavor to the bread. It is perishable and should be used within a short period....

Proofing Yeast...

Properly proofing yeast ensures its viability and activates its fermentation potential. This step is crucial for achieving an optimal rise in your bread....

Water Temperature...

The water used to proof yeast should be at a specific temperature range, typically between 100°F to

110°F (38°C to 43°C). Too hot or too cold water can inhibit yeast activity....

Sugar or Honey...

Adding a small amount of sugar or honey to the proofing liquid provides yeast with an initial source of food, encouraging activation....

Foam Formation...

After a few minutes, the yeast mixture should begin to foam and bubble. This indicates that the yeast is active and ready to be incorporated into the dough....

By understanding the characteristics and activation process of yeast, you'll be able to harness its power to create beautifully risen and flavorful breads. In the next chapters, we'll explore the fermentation process and kneading techniques, building on this foundational knowledge....

Chapter 4: Understanding the Fermentation Process...

Fermentation is a transformative stage in bread making, where yeast and beneficial bacteria work together to develop flavor, texture, and structure. Mastering this process is essential for creating exceptional loaves of bread....

The Role of Fermentation...

During fermentation, yeast consumes sugars in the dough, producing carbon dioxide and alcohol. This action leavens the bread, creating a light and airy crumb. Additionally, beneficial bacteria contribute to the development of complex flavors....

Extended Fermentation...

Allowing the dough to ferment over an extended period, often in the refrigerator, enhances flavor and texture. This slow, cold fermentation process leads to a more nuanced and aromatic final product....

Temperature and Time...

Controlling the temperature and duration of fermentation is key to achieving the desired results in your bread....

Ambient Temperature...

Warmer environments accelerate fermentation, resulting in a quicker rise and a slightly different flavor profile. Cooler temperatures slow down the process, allowing for more flavor development....

Refrigeration...

Refrigeration slows down fermentation, providing an opportunity for flavors to deepen and mature. It also offers flexibility in your baking schedule....

Autolyse: Resting the Dough...

Autolyse is a technique that involves allowing the dough to rest after the initial mixing and before the addition of salt. This period of rest allows the flour to fully hydrate, resulting in improved gluten development and a smoother texture....

Fermentation Techniques for Sourdough...

In sourdough baking, wild yeast and lactic acid bacteria drive the fermentation process. Understanding the unique characteristics of sourdough cultures and how to maintain them is essential for successful sourdough bread....

By mastering the principles of fermentation, you'll have the ability to manipulate flavor profiles and textures to create bread that suits your personal taste preferences....

Chapter 5: Kneading Techniques for Perfect Dough...

Kneading is a crucial step in bread making that develops the gluten structure, providing the necessary support for the dough to rise. There are various techniques you can employ to achieve optimal results....

Hand Kneading...

Hand kneading involves a rhythmic motion of folding, pressing, and turning the dough. This process allows you to feel the changes in the dough's texture and elasticity....

Stand Mixer with Dough Hook...

A stand mixer equipped with a dough hook is a convenient tool for kneading, especially for large batches. It automates the process, allowing for consistent and thorough gluten development....

Stretch and Fold Technique...

This no-knead technique involves gently stretching and folding the dough at intervals during the bulk fermentation stage. It promotes gluten development without the need for extensive kneading....

Windowpane Test...

The windowpane test is a reliable way to determine if the dough has been adequately kneaded. Gently stretch a small piece of dough between your fingers. If it forms a thin, translucent membrane without tearing, the gluten is well-developed....

Adjusting Kneading Time...

The duration of kneading varies depending on factors such as flour type, hydration level, and desired bread texture. Observing the dough's progress and making adjustments as needed is crucial for achieving the desired result....

By mastering the art of kneading, you'll be able to consistently produce bread with a desirable texture and structure. In the following chapters, we will explore the art of shaping and proofing, as well as the precise details of baking time and temperature....

Chapter 6: The Art of Shaping and Proofing...

Shaping and proofing are critical steps that contribute to the final appearance and texture of your bread. Mastering these techniques will elevate your baking to a professional level....

Shaping Techniques...

Properly shaping the dough ensures that it maintains its structure during the final rise and baking....

Boule (Round Loaf)...

To shape a boule, gently flatten the dough into a circle. Fold the edges towards the center, creating tension on the surface. Rotate and repeat until a taut ball forms....

Batard (Oblong Loaf)...

For a batard, start with a rectangle of dough. Fold the top third towards the center, pressing to seal. Then fold the bottom third up and seal. Roll and taper the ends....

Baguette...

Begin by flattening the dough into a rectangle. Fold the top and bottom edges towards the center, then roll up tightly, sealing the seam....

Ciabatta...

Maintain a wet dough and handle it gently to preserve air bubbles. Shape into a rectangle, avoiding excess deflation. Use a peel to transfer onto the baking surface....

Final Proofing...

The final proof, or second rise, is essential for achieving a light and airy crumb in your bread....

Temperature and Humidity...

Controlled conditions are crucial for a successful final proof. Slightly warmer and more humid environments encourage a steady rise....

Visual Cues...

Look for signs of fermentation, such as increased volume and a slightly domed shape. Be cautious not to overproof, which can lead to collapsed loaves....

Fingertip Test...

Gently press the dough with your fingertip. If it springs back slowly, it's ready. If it springs back quickly, it needs more time. If it doesn't spring back at all, it's overproofed....

Scoring the Dough...

Before baking, make deliberate cuts, or scores, on the surface of the dough. This allows for controlled expansion and creates an attractive appearance....

Tools for Scoring...

A sharp blade or a specialized scoring tool can be used. Hold the tool at a slight angle and make swift, confident cuts....

Creative Scoring...

Experiment with different patterns and designs to add a personal touch to your loaves....

By mastering the art of shaping and proofing, you'll be able to craft visually appealing and perfectly textured breads. In the next chapter, we will explore the precise details of baking temperature and timing to bring your creations to perfection....

Chapter 7: Baking: Temperature and Timing...

Baking is the final crucial step in the bread-making process, where the dough transforms into a golden, fragrant loaf. Understanding the nuances of temperature and timing is key to achieving bakery-quality results....

Preheating Your Oven...

Properly preheating your oven ensures that the bread receives the initial burst of heat needed for a good rise and crust development....

Standard Baking Temperatures...

Most bread recipes call for an initial high temperature (around 450°F/232°C) to create steam and promote oven spring. This is typically followed by a lower baking temperature to ensure even cooking....

Using a Baking Stone or Dutch Oven...

Placing a baking stone or a Dutch oven in the oven while it preheats can help replicate the intense heat of a professional bread oven....

Steam for a Crisp Crust...

Introducing steam into the oven at the beginning of the baking process creates a humid environment, allowing the crust to expand before setting....

Methods for Steam...

You can achieve steam by placing a pan of boiling water on the bottom rack of the oven or by spritzing the dough with water before placing it in the oven....

Monitoring and Rotating...

Keeping an eye on your bread as it bakes allows you to make adjustments if needed....

Rotation...

Rotate the bread halfway through the baking time to ensure even browning....

Oven Hot Spots...

Be aware of any hot spots in your oven, which can cause uneven baking. Adjusting the position of your bread may be necessary....

Achieving the Desired Doneness...

Determining when your bread is fully baked involves a combination of visual and auditory cues....

Visual Cues...

Look for a deep, golden-brown crust. The bread should sound hollow when tapped on the bottom....

Internal Temperature...

For added precision, you can use an instant-read thermometer. The internal temperature of fully baked bread should register between 190°F to 210°F (88°C to 99°C)....

Cooling and Resting...

Allowing the bread to cool properly is essential for achieving the best texture and flavor....

Cooling Rack...

Transfer the bread to a wire rack to cool. Elevating it allows for air circulation, preventing condensation....

Resting Time...

Resist the urge to slice into the bread immediately. Allowing it to rest for at least an hour ensures that the interior sets properly....

By understanding the interplay of temperature and timing, you'll be able to consistently produce breads with a crisp crust, tender crumb, and optimal flavor. In the next chapter, we'll explore techniques for adding flavors and enhancements to your bread, allowing you to customize your creations to your liking....

Chapter 8: Adding Flavors and Enhancements...

Elevate your bread-making skills by incorporating a variety of flavors and enhancements. These additions can transform a simple loaf into a culinary masterpiece....

Herbs and Spices...

Experiment with a wide range of herbs and spices to infuse your bread with unique and aromatic flavors....

Fresh Herbs...

Chopped fresh herbs like rosemary, thyme, or basil can be folded into the dough during the mixing process....

Spices and Seasonings...

Ground spices such as cinnamon, nutmeg, or cumin can be added for a hint of warmth and complexity....

Nuts and Seeds...

Nuts and seeds provide texture, crunch, and added nutritional value to your bread....

Toasting for Depth of Flavor...

Toasting nuts and seeds before incorporating them into the dough enhances their nuttiness and aroma....

Proper Distribution...

Evenly distribute nuts and seeds throughout the dough to ensure every slice is filled with deliciousness....

Fruits and Vegetables...

Incorporating fruits and vegetables can add natural sweetness, moisture, and color to your bread....

Dried Fruits...

Chopped dried fruits like apricots, cranberries, or figs can be soaked and folded into the dough....

Grated Vegetables...

Carrots, zucchini, or sweet potatoes can be grated and folded into the dough for added moisture and flavor....

Cheese and Dairy...

Cheese and dairy products bring richness and creaminess to your bread, creating a luxurious eating experience....

Grated Cheese...

Sharp cheddar, Parmesan, or Gruyère can be folded into the dough for a savory twist....

Yogurt or Buttermilk...

Substituting a portion of the water with yogurt or buttermilk adds tanginess and tenderness to the crumb....

Sweeteners...

Adding sweeteners enhances the flavor profile of your bread, making it suitable for both savory and dessert applications....

Honey, Maple Syrup, or Molasses...

These natural sweeteners impart depth and complexity to the flavor of your bread....

Adjusting for Sweetness...

Experiment with the amount of sweetener to achieve your desired level of sweetness....

By incorporating these flavor-enhancing elements, you'll have the opportunity to create breads that cater to a wide range of tastes and preferences. In the following chapters, we'll explore specialty breads, troubleshooting common issues, and delving into gluten-free and alternative grain baking....

Chapter 9: Specialty Breads: Beyond the Basics...

Dive into the world of specialty breads, where unique ingredients and techniques result in exceptional and distinctive loaves....

Focaccia...

Originating from Italy, focaccia is a flat, oven-baked bread known for its dimpled surface and aromatic toppings....

Olive Oil Infusion...

Generously drizzle olive oil on the dough before baking to achieve a crisp crust and a moist, flavorful crumb....

Toppings and Herbs...

Experiment with toppings like cherry tomatoes, olives, rosemary, or caramelized onions for added flavor and visual appeal....

Challah...

This Jewish braided bread is rich, slightly sweet, and has a beautiful golden crust....

Enriched Dough...

Challah dough contains eggs and honey, giving it a tender, golden crumb and a slightly sweet flavor....

Braiding Techniques...

Explore various braiding patterns to create intricate and stunning designs....

Brioche...

Known for its high butter content, brioche is a decadently rich and tender bread that's perfect for both sweet and savory applications....

Incorporating Butter...

Slowly incorporating softened butter into the dough during mixing creates a lusciously soft crumb....

Shaping Options...

Brioche can be shaped into loaves, rolls, or even intricate pastries like brioche à tête....

Bagels...

Bagels have a chewy interior and a shiny, firm crust, achieved through a unique boiling and baking process....

Boiling the Dough...

Boiling the shaped bagels in water before baking sets the crust and gives them their distinctive texture....

Toppings and Fillings...

Sesame seeds, poppy seeds, or even savory fillings like cheese or everything seasoning can be added for extra flavor....

Sourdough Varieties...

Explore the world of sourdough beyond the basic loaf with specialty variations like olive sourdough, walnut sourdough, or multigrain sourdough....

Incorporating Add-Ins...

Fold in chopped olives, toasted nuts, or a mixture of grains to add texture and flavor to your sourdough....

Extended Fermentation...

Allowing the dough to ferment for an extended period enhances the complexity of the flavor....

By delving into specialty breads, you'll have the opportunity to explore unique flavors and techniques that will impress both yourself and your guests. In the next chapter, we'll address common troubleshooting issues that may arise during the bread-making process....

Chapter 10: Troubleshooting Common Bread Baking Issues...

Even experienced bakers encounter challenges from time to time. Understanding and addressing common issues will help you overcome hurdles and achieve consistent success in your bread making....

Overproofing...

Overproofed dough may result in a collapsed, dense loaf with a gummy texture....

Prevention:...

Monitor the dough closely during the final proofing stage....

Use the fingertip test to gauge readiness....

Underproofing...

Underproofed dough may lead to a dense, overly chewy crumb....

Solution:...

Extend the final proofing time as needed....

Ensure the dough has doubled in size and holds its shape....

Poor Rise...

Insufficient rise may be caused by inactive yeast, improper fermentation, or cool room temperatures....

Solutions:...

Verify the viability of your yeast....

Ensure adequate fermentation time, adjusting for room temperature....

Uneven Crumb Structure...

Inconsistent crumb may result from uneven mixing or shaping....

Solutions:...

Thoroughly mix ingredients, ensuring even distribution....

Pay attention to uniform shaping techniques....

Gummy or Wet Interior...

A gummy interior may be caused by excess moisture, underbaking, or insufficient cooling....

Solutions:...

Adjust hydration levels to avoid overly wet dough....

Bake until the internal temperature reaches the desired range....

Dense Texture...

Dense bread may occur due to insufficient gluten development, improper shaping, or expired yeast....

Solutions:...

Adequately knead the dough for proper gluten structure....

Ensure that your yeast is fresh and active....

Pale Crust...

A pale crust may result from insufficient oven temperature or inadequate baking time....

Solutions:...

Preheat your oven thoroughly to ensure proper heat transfer....

Extend baking time as needed, watching for desired coloration....

Cracked Crust...

A cracked crust may occur due to rapid oven spring or uneven shaping....

Solutions:...

Score the dough to allow for controlled expansion....

Ensure even shaping to distribute tension....

Flat Loaf...

A flat loaf may be caused by overmixing, underproofing, or inadequate oven spring....

Solutions:...

Avoid excessive mixing to preserve structure....

Allow for sufficient final proofing before baking....

By recognizing and addressing these common issues, you'll be equipped to troubleshoot and refine your bread-making process. In the next chapter, we'll explore the world of gluten-free and alternative grain baking, catering to a wider range of dietary preferences....

Chapter 11: Gluten-Free and Alternative Grain Baking...

For those with gluten sensitivities or dietary preferences, exploring gluten-free and alternative grain baking opens up a world of delicious possibilities....

Gluten-Free Flours...

A variety of gluten-free flours can be used as alternatives to wheat flour, each offering unique textures and flavors....

Almond Flour...

Rich in healthy fats, almond flour lends a moist and nutty flavor to baked goods....

Coconut Flour...

High in fiber and low in carbohydrates, coconut flour provides a unique texture and mild coconut flavor....

Rice Flour...

Milled from either white or brown rice, rice flour offers a neutral flavor and fine texture....

Nut and Seed Flours...

Ground nuts and seeds can be used to create flour alternatives with distinct flavors and added nutritional benefits....

Hazelnut Flour...

With a rich, toasty flavor, hazelnut flour adds depth to baked goods....

Sunflower Seed Flour...

Ground sunflower seeds offer a nutty taste and a unique texture....

Alternative Grains...

Exploring alternative grains introduces a wide range of flavors and textures to your baked goods....

Quinoa Flour...

Rich in protein and nutrients, quinoa flour provides a nutty flavor and a slightly dense texture....

Teff Flour...

Originating from Ethiopia, teff flour is known for its earthy flavor and fine texture....

Binder and Leavening Agents...

In gluten-free baking, it's crucial to incorporate binders and leavening agents to achieve the desired texture....

Xanthan Gum...

Xanthan gum acts as a binder, providing structure to gluten-free baked goods....

Baking Powder and Baking Soda...

These leavening agents help achieve a light and airy texture in your gluten-free creations....

Hydration Adjustments...

Gluten-free flours may absorb moisture differently than wheat flour. Adjusting hydration levels can lead to better results....

By exploring gluten-free and alternative grain baking, you'll be able to cater to a wider range of dietary preferences while still creating delicious and satisfying bread. In the next chapter, we'll delve into the art of sourdough baking, from cultivating a starter to mastering the intricacies of the process....

Chapter 12: Sourdough Mastery: From Starter to Loaf...

Sourdough baking is an ancient and rewarding tradition, resulting in flavorful, naturally leavened bread. Mastering the process involves understanding the nuances of creating and maintaining a sourdough starter....

Creating a Sourdough Starter...

A sourdough starter is a living culture of wild yeast and bacteria that provides leavening for your bread....

Flour and Water...

Mix equal parts flour and water to create a thick, pancake-like batter. Allow it to ferment in a warm environment....

Feeding the Starter...

Regular feedings of fresh flour and water are essential to maintain a healthy and active starter....

Starter Hydration Levels...

Adjusting the ratio of flour to water can influence the activity and consistency of your starter....

Starter Maintenance...

Proper care and feeding of your starter ensure its vitality and flavor contribution to your bread....

Feeding Schedule...

Establish a regular feeding schedule to keep your starter active. This may vary based on room temperature and the type of flour used....

Temperature Considerations...

Temperature significantly impacts the fermentation rate of your starter. Cooler environments result in slower fermentation, while warmer temperatures accelerate the process....

Incorporating the Starter into Your Dough...

Once your starter is robust and active, it becomes the leavening agent for your sourdough bread....

Autolyse and Mixing...

Allowing the flour and water to rest before incorporating the starter improves gluten development and dough consistency....

Bulk Fermentation and Folds...

During bulk fermentation, perform periodic folds to strengthen the dough and distribute the starter....

Final Proofing...

Allow the shaped dough to undergo final proofing until it reaches the desired level of readiness....

Baking Sourdough Bread...

Baking with a sourdough starter requires attentiveness to achieve optimal results....

Scoring and Steam...

Score the surface of the dough to control expansion and create an attractive pattern. Introduce steam for a crisp crust....

Oven Spring and Doneness...

Monitor the dough as it bakes to ensure proper oven spring and achieve the desired level of doneness....

By mastering the art of sourdough baking, you'll have the opportunity to create bread with a distinctive, complex flavor profile and a beautifully textured crumb. In the next chapter, we'll explore the techniques of artisanal bread making, including advanced shaping and flavor development....

Chapter 13: Artisanal Bread: Techniques for the Pros...

Artisanal bread making involves advanced techniques and a deep understanding of the bread-making process. Elevate your baking skills with these intricate methods....

Pre-Ferments...

Pre-ferments are pre-made doughs or batters that undergo fermentation before being incorporated into the final dough....

Poolish...

A wet, batter-like pre-ferment with equal parts flour and water, poolish adds depth of flavor and improved texture to the bread....

Biga...

A stiffer, drier pre-ferment with a higher proportion of flour, biga contributes a mild, nutty flavor and a chewy crumb....

Advanced Shaping Techniques...

Artisanal bread often showcases intricate shaping methods for distinctive visual appeal....

Batard with Ears...

Achieve a rustic, ear-like shape by creating tension during shaping and scoring....

Couronne Bordelaise...

Craft a crown-shaped bread by delicately folding and shaping the dough....

Flavor Development...

Artisanal breads often incorporate extended fermentation or unique ingredients for enhanced flavor....

Retarded Fermentation...

Refrigerating the dough for an extended period allows for complex flavor development....

Additions like Grains and Seeds...

Incorporate whole grains, seeds, or cereals to impart texture and a nutty flavor....

Professional Scoring Techniques...

Elaborate scoring patterns can elevate the visual presentation of your bread....

Wheat Sheaf...

Create an intricate pattern resembling a sheaf of wheat to showcase your skill....

Fougasse...

Craft a leaf-shaped bread with precise, strategic cuts....

Advanced Baking Methods...

Artisanal bread making may involve unconventional baking techniques....

Steam Injection...

Injecting steam into the oven creates a professional-grade, crisp crust....

Hearth Baking...

Using a baking stone or a dedicated hearth oven simulates

the intense heat of a traditional bread oven....

By incorporating these advanced techniques, you'll have the opportunity to create bread that not only delights the palate but also dazzles the eyes. In the final chapter, we'll explore how bread can be a culinary canvas, inviting you to experiment with creative recipes and flavor combinations....

Chapter 14: Bread as a Culinary Canvas: Creative Recipes...

Embrace your inner culinary artist and use bread as a versatile canvas for a wide range of creative and innovative recipes....

Stuffed Breads...

Experiment with fillings and create flavorful, surprise-filled loaves....

Spinach and Feta Stuffed Bread...

Combine sautéed spinach and crumbled feta for a savory filling....

Cinnamon Sugar Swirl Bread...

Create a sweet treat with a cinnamon-sugar filling for a delightful twist on traditional bread....

Artisanal Toppings...

Elevate your bread with unique and flavorful toppings....

Everything Bagel Topping...

Coat your bread with a mixture of sesame seeds, poppy seeds, garlic, onion, and salt for a burst of flavor....

Olive Tapenade and Herbed Butter...

Spread a mixture of olives, capers, and herbs over warm bread for a Mediterranean-inspired delight....

Bread Bowls and Dips...

Transform loaves into edible serving vessels for savory dips and spreads....

Spinach and Artichoke Dip...

Hollow out a round loaf, fill it with a creamy spinach and artichoke dip, and bake for a delectable appetizer....

Cheese Fondue Bread Bowl...

Create a warm, gooey cheese fondue inside a hollowed-out bread loaf for a crowd-pleasing party dish....

Sweet Breads and Desserts...

Explore the sweeter side of bread-making with decadent recipes....

Chocolate Babka...

Swirl layers of chocolate and cinnamon within the dough for a rich, indulgent treat....

Fruit and Nut Braid...

Weave together a mixture of dried fruits and nuts for a delightful, sweet bread....

Global Flavors...

Draw inspiration from cuisines around the world to infuse unique flavors into your bread....

Focaccia di Recco...

Hailing from Italy, this thin, cheese-filled focaccia is a delightful combination of crisp and chewy textures....

Pão de Queijo Rolls...

These Brazilian cheese bread rolls are naturally gluten-free and feature a chewy interior and a crispy crust....

By exploring creative recipes, you'll have the opportunity to take your bread-making skills to new heights, impressing friends and family with your culinary ingenuity. This concludes our journey through the art and science of bread making. May your kitchen be filled with the warm, inviting aroma of freshly baked bread for years to come. Happy baking!...

Chapter 15: The Bread Maker's Journey...

As you reach the final chapter of this comprehensive guide to bread making, it's important to reflect on your journey and the knowledge you've acquired....

Honing Your Craft...

Bread making is a craft that rewards patience, practice, and a lifelong commitment to learning....

Record Your Experiences...

Maintain a baking journal to document your recipes, observations, and successes. This will help you refine your skills over time....

Seek Inspiration...

Continue to explore new recipes, techniques, and ingredients to keep your passion for bread making alive....

Sharing Your Creations...

One of the joys of bread making is sharing your delicious creations with others....

Host Bread Workshops...

Consider hosting workshops or classes to share your expertise and

passion with friends, family, or
your community....

Bake for Special Occasions...

Bread makes a thoughtful and
memorable gift for holidays,
birthdays, or other special
occasions....

Sustainable Practices...

Embrace sustainable practices to
minimize waste and reduce your
carbon footprint....

Sourdough Starter Care...

Share your sourdough starter with
others to promote sustainability
and a sense of community....

Reduce Food Waste...

Repurpose stale bread into croutons, breadcrumbs, or bread pudding to minimize waste....

A Lifelong Journey...

Remember that bread making is a journey, not a destination. There is always more to learn and explore....

Adapt and Experiment...

Be open to adaptation and experimentation. Innovation often leads to remarkable discoveries in the world of bread....

Pass It On...

Pass down your bread-making knowledge to future generations, ensuring that this timeless tradition endures....

As you conclude your exploration
of bread making, know that you
have not only acquired a valuable
skill but also become part of a
global community that cherishes
the art and science of bread.
Continue to knead, shape, and
bake with love, and let the aroma
of freshly baked bread fill your
home for generations to come.
Your journey as a bread maker is a
lifelong adventure filled with
warmth, flavor, and endless
possibilities....

9 7 9 8 8 7 4 1 9 4 8 8 8